KETO DIET POULTRY AND OTHER MEAT

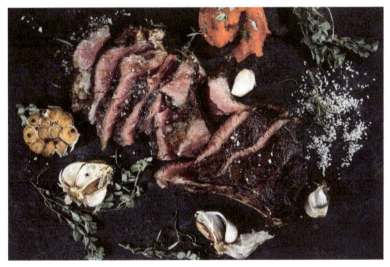

RECIPES

Katie Hudson

Table of Contents

POULTRY 9

    Amazing Sour Cream Chicken 10

    Ethiopian Doro Watt Chicken 11

    Mexican Chicken Soup 13

    Delicious Southwest Chicken 15

    Flavors Peanut Butter Chicken 17

    Easy Salsa Chicken 19

    Greek Lemon Chicken 21

    Easy Chicken Noodles 23

    Orange Chicken 25

    Delicious BBQ Chicken 27

    Parmesan Chicken Rice 29

    Queso Chicken Tacos 31

    Easy Mexican Chicken 32

    Mustard Mushroom Chicken 33

    Herb Chicken Breasts 35

Balsamic Chicken 37

Creamy Chicken Penne 39

Tasty Chicken Fajita Pasta 41

Moist & Juicy Chicken Breast 43

Asian Chicken 45

Flavorful Chicken Casserole 47

Chicken Orzo 49

Garlic Herb Roasted Pepper Chicken 51

Slow Cook Turkey Breast 53

Simple Chicken & Mushrooms 55

Lemon Herb Chicken 56

Creamy Chicken Curry 58

Taco Chicken 60

Butter Chicken 61

Spicy Chili Chicken 62

Pesto Chicken 64

Rosemary Turkey Breast 65

Garlic Olive Chicken 66

Delicious Chickpea Chicken 68

Chicken Kale Soup 70

Creamy Italian Chicken 72

Chicken and Vegetables 73

Chicken Gyros 74

Crockpot Creamy Salsa Chicken 76

Pizza Casserole 77

Moist and Spicy Pulled Chicken Breast 78

Whole Roasted Chicken 80

Simple Chicken Chili 82

Chicken in Salsa Verde 84

Egg Casserole with Italian Cheeses, Sun-Dried Tomatoes, and Herbs 86

Egg and Cheese Casserole with Chayote Squash 87

Scrambled Eggs with Smoked Salmon 89

PORK & LAMB 92

Mouth-Watering Minced Pork Zucchini Lasagna 93

Beautiful BBQ Ribs 95

Gorgeous Coconut Turmeric Pork Curry 97

Kalua Pork.. 99

Tasty Cuban Mojo Pork 100

Slow Cooker Pork Loin 102

Green Chili Pork 104

Thai Curried Pork 106

Chinese 5-Spice Pork Ribs..108

Pork Stew with Oyster Mushrooms 110

Paprika Pork Tenderloin 112

Pork Carnitas 114

Lemongrass Coconut Pulled Pork............................... 116

Pork Loin Roast with Onion Gravy 118

Lime Pork Chops..120

Chili Pulled Pork 122

Ranch Pork Chops 124

Delicious Coconut Pork 125

Spicy Adobo Pulled Pork 127

Tasty Pork Tacos 128

Lamb Provençal 130

Greek Style Lamb Shanks..132

Lamb with Mint & Green Beans..................................134

Delicious Balsamic Lamb Chops 136

Succulent Lamb 137

Tarragon Lamb & Beans...139

Apricot Pulled Pork.. 141

Tantalizing Pork Chops with Cumin Butter and Garlic 142

New Mexico Carne Adovada..144

Smoky Pork with Cabbage..146

Simple Roasted Pork Shoulder...................................148

Flavors Pork Chops...149

Pork Loin with Peanut Sauce 151

POULTRY

Amazing Sour Cream Chicken

Preparation Time: 15 minutes

Cooking Time: 6 hours

Servings: 4

Ingredients:

1 cup of sour cream

½ cup of chicken stock

1 can of diced green chilies and tomatoes

1 batch of taco seasoning

2 pounds of chicken breast

Directions:

Put all the items to the slow cooker. Cook on low for 6 hours. Divide onto plates and serve.

Nutrition:

Calories: 262 Fat: 13 g Fiber: 2.5 g

Protein: 32 g Carbs: 23 g

Ethiopian Doro Watt Chicken

Preparation Time: 35 minutes
Cooking Time: 8 hours
Servings: 6
Ingredients:
1 tsp chili powder
1 tsp sweet paprika
½ tsp ground ginger
1 tbsp salt
1 tsp ground coriander
1/8 tsp ground cardamom
1/8 tsp allspice
1/8 tsp fenugreek powder
1/8 tsp nutmeg
1 whole chicken, sliced into different parts
½ c. butter
1 clove of garlic, minced
1/2 c. water
2 large onions, chopped

8 hard-boiled eggs

Directions:

Combine the first 9 items in a bowl. Use this spice mix and rub it on the chicken parts. Marinate within 30 minutes in the fridge.

Take the butter in the crockpot and add the onion and garlic. Take the chicken pieces. Arrange the hard-boiled eggs randomly on top of the chicken.

Pour water, then cook on low within 8 hours.

Nutrition:

Calories: 315 Carbohydrates:4g Protein: 19g

Fat: 25g Sugar: 0g Sodium: 698mg Fiber: 0.8g

Mexican Chicken Soup

Preparation Time: 15 minutes
Cooking Time: 8 hours
Servings: 6
Ingredients:
6 cups chicken broth

4 teaspoons garlic

0.25 cups jalapeno

1 tablespoon cumin

1 tablespoon chili powder

0.5 cups cilantro

2 tablespoons lime juice

1.5 cups carrots

0.66 cups onion

0.5 cups Roma tomato

0.75 cups tomato juice

1 teaspoon coriander

2 teaspoons sea salt

4 cups chicken breast

Directions:

Chop herbs and vegetables. Put everything in the cooker. Low cook for 8 hours. Serve.

Nutrition:

Calories 296 Fat 16 g

Protein 27 g Carbs 10 g

Delicious Southwest Chicken

Preparation Time: 10 minutes
Cooking Time: 6 hours
Servings: 8
Ingredients:

4 chicken breasts, skinless & boneless

1 tsp cumin powder

1 tbsp chili powder

2 garlic cloves, minced

1 small onion, chopped

4 oz can green chilies, diced

15 oz can corn, drained

15 oz can black beans, drained & rinsed

1 cup of salsa

1 cup chicken broth

1/2 tsp salt

Directions:

Add all ingredients into the cooking pot and stir well.

Cover instant pot aura with lid.

Select slow cook mode and cook on LOW for 6 hours.

Remove chicken from pot and shred using a fork.

Return shredded chicken to the cooking pot and stir well.

Serve over cooked rice.

Nutrition:

Calories 256 Fat 6.6 g

Carbohydrates 23.9 g

Sugar

Flavors Peanut Butter Chicken

Preparation Time: 10 minutes
Cooking Time: 8 hours
Servings: 4
Ingredients:

3 lbs chicken breasts, bone-in & skinless

3 tbsp maple syrup

1/2 tbsp rice wine vinegar

1 tbsp coarse whole grain mustard

1 tbsp garlic, minced

2 tbsp chili garlic sauce

1/2 cup soy sauce

1/2 lime juice

1/4 cup peanut butter

Pepper

salt

Directions:

Season chicken with pepper and salt and place into the cooking pot. Mix together remaining ingredients and pour over chicken in the cooking pot. Cover instant pot aura with lid.

Select slow cook mode and cook on LOW for 8 hours.

Remove chicken from pot and shred using a fork.

Serve and enjoy.

Nutrition:

Calories 806 Fat 33.5 g Carbohydrates 17.1 g

Sugar 11.1 g

Easy Salsa Chicken

Preparation Time: 10 minutes
Cooking Time: 3 hours
Servings: 4
Ingredients:
2 1/2 lbs chicken breasts, bone-in & skinless
1 1/2 cups salsa
3 tsp ranch seasoning
Pepper
Salt
Directions:
Add 1/2 cup salsa into the cooking pot then place chicken on top of salsa. Season with ranch seasoning, pepper, and salt.
Pour remaining salsa over chicken in the cooking pot.
Cover instant pot aura with lid. Select slow cook mode and cook on HIGH for 3 hours. Remove chicken from pot and shred using a fork.
Serve and enjoy.

Nutrition:

Calories 573 Fat 21.2 g Carbohydrates 6.1 g

Sugar 3 g Protein 83.5 g

Cholesterol 252 mg

Greek Lemon Chicken

Preparation Time: 10 minutes
Cooking Time: 6 hours
Servings: 4
Ingredients:
4 chicken breasts, skinless & boneless
3 tbsp parsley, chopped
1 cup chicken broth
1 tbsp lemon zest
1/4 cup lemon juice
2 tsp dried oregano
1 tbsp garlic, minced
1 tsp kosher salt

Directions:
Add all ingredients into the cooking pot and mix well.
Cover instant pot aura with lid.
Select slow cook mode and cook on LOW for 6 hours.
Serve and enjoy.

Nutrition:
Calories 296 Fat 11.3 g

Carbohydrates 1.7 g
Sugar 0.6 g
Protein 43.8 g
Cholesterol 130 mg

Easy Chicken Noodles

Preparation Time: 10 minutes
Cooking Time: 6 hours 30 minutes
Servings: 8
Ingredients:
4 chicken breasts, skinless & boneless
12 oz egg noodles
14.5 oz chicken broth
21 oz cream of chicken soup
Pepper
Salt
Directions:
Add chicken, broth, soup, pepper, and salt into the cooking pot and stir well.
Cover instant pot aura with lid.
Select slow cook mode and cook on HIGH for 6 hours.
Remove chicken from pot and shred using a fork, return shredded chicken to the pot and stir well.
Add noodles into the cooking pot and cook for 30 minutes more.

Stir well and serve.

Nutrition:

Calories 273

Fat 10.9 g

Carbohydrates 16.2 g

Sugar 0.7 g

Protein 25.9 g

Cholesterol 83 mg

Orange Chicken

Preparation Time: 10 minutes

Cooking Time: 7 hours

Servings: 6

Ingredients:

1 lb chicken breasts, skinless & boneless

2 tbsp soy sauce

1 cup sweet orange marmalade

1 cup BBQ sauce

Directions:

Add all ingredients into the cooking pot and stir well.

Cover instant pot aura with lid.

Select slow cook mode and cook on LOW for 7 hours.

Remove chicken from pot and shred using a fork, return shredded chicken to the pot and stir well.

Serve and enjoy.

Nutrition:

Calories 342

Fat 5.7 g

Carbohydrates 50.2 g

Sugar 43 g
Protein 22.2 g
Cholesterol 67 mg

Delicious BBQ Chicken

Preparation Time: 10 minutes
Cooking Time: 4 hours
Servings: 8
Ingredients:

3 lbs chicken breasts, skinless & boneless

2 tbsp brown sugar

1 tbsp Worcestershire sauce

1 tbsp olive oil

1/2 onion, grated

1 1/2 cups BBQ sauce

Directions:

Add all ingredients into the cooking pot and stir well.

Cover instant pot aura with lid.

Select slow cook mode and cook on HIGH for 4 hours.

Remove chicken from pot and shred using a fork, return shredded chicken to the pot and stir well.

Serve and enjoy.

Nutrition:

Calories 422 Fat 14.5 g

Carbohydrates 20.2 g

Sugar 15.1 g Protein 49.3 g

Cholesterol 151 mg

Parmesan Chicken Rice

Preparation Time: 10 minutes

Cooking Time: 4 hours

Servings: 6

Ingredients:

4 chicken breasts, skinless & boneless

1/4 cup parmesan cheese, grated

1 cup of rice

1 3/4 cups milk

21 oz can cream of chicken soup

Pepper

Salt

Directions:

Season chicken with pepper and salt and place into the cooking pot.

Mix together rice, milk, and soup and pour over chicken and top with parmesan cheese.

Cover instant pot aura with lid.

Select slow cook mode and cook on HIGH for 4 hours.

Remove chicken from pot and chop, return chicken to the pot and stir well.

Serve and enjoy.

Nutrition:

Calories 453 Fat 16.7 g

Carbohydrates 35.6 g Sugar 3.8 g

Protein 38.2 g Cholesterol 107 mg

Queso Chicken Tacos

Preparation Time: 10 minutes
Cooking Time: 4 hours
Servings: 8
Ingredients:
2 lbs chicken breasts, boneless & skinless

1 1/2 cups Mexican cheese dip

10 oz can Rotel

1 oz taco seasoning

Directions:
Add all ingredients into the cooking pot and stir well.

Cover instant pot aura with lid.

Select slow cook mode and cook on LOW for 4-6 hours.

Remove chicken from pot and shred using a fork, return shredded chicken to the pot and stir well.

Serve and enjoy.

Nutrition:
Calories 349 Fat 17.8 g Carbohydrates 4.7 g

Sugar 0.9 g Protein 39.5 g Cholesterol 120 mg

Easy Mexican Chicken

Preparation Time: 10 minutes

Cooking Time: 6 hours

Servings: 6

Ingredients:

2 lbs chicken breasts, boneless & skinless

1/3 cup chicken stock

1 oz taco seasoning

2 cups salsa

Directions:

Add all ingredients into the cooking pot and stir well.

Cover instant pot aura with lid.

Select slow cook mode and cook on LOW for 6 hours.

Remove chicken from pot and shred using a fork, return shredded chicken to the pot and stir well.

Serve and enjoy.

Nutrition:

Calories 321 Fat 11.9 g Carbohydrates 6.2 g

Sugar 2.7 g Protein 45.7 g

Mustard Mushroom Chicken

Preparation Time: 10 minutes
Cooking Time: 6 hours
Servings: 4
Ingredients:

4 chicken thighs, bone-in & skin-on

1 tsp garlic, minced

1 tsp grainy mustard

8 oz mushrooms, sliced

10.5 oz cream of mushroom soup

Pepper

Salt

Directions:

Season chicken with pepper and salt and place into the cooking pot.

Mix together remaining ingredients and pour over chicken.

Cover instant pot aura with lid.

Select slow cook mode and cook on LOW for 6 hours. Serve and enjoy.

Nutrition:

Calories 324 Fat 13.3 g Carbohydrates 4.7 g

Sugar 1.5 g Protein 44.8 g Cholesterol 130 mg

Herb Chicken Breasts

Preparation Time: 10 minutes

Cooking Time: 5 hours

Servings: 6

Ingredients:

6 chicken breasts, boneless & skinless

1/3 cup dry white wine

1 garlic clove, crushed

1 tsp thyme, chopped

2 tsp fresh oregano, chopped

Pepper

Salt

Directions:

Season chicken with pepper and salt and place into the cooking pot. Mix together remaining ingredients and pour over chicken.

Cover instant pot aura with lid. Select slow cook mode and cook on LOW for 5 hours.

Serve and enjoy.

Nutrition:

Calories 291 Fat 10.9 g Carbohydrates 1 g
Sugar 0.1 g Protein 42.4 g Cholesterol 130 mg

Balsamic Chicken

Preparation Time: 10 minutes

Cooking Time: 4 hours

Servings: 10

Ingredients:

4 chicken breasts, boneless & skinless

1/2 tsp thyme

1 tsp dried rosemary

1 tsp dried basil

1 tsp dried oregano

1 tbsp olive oil

1/2 cup balsamic vinegar

4 garlic cloves

1 onion, sliced

30 oz can tomatoes, diced

Pepper

Salt

Directions:

Season chicken with pepper and salt and place into the cooking pot.

Mix together remaining ingredients and pour over chicken.

Cover instant pot aura with lid.

Select slow cook mode and cook on HIGH for 4 hours.

Serve and enjoy.

Nutrition:

Calories 151 Fat 5.8 g

Carbohydrates 6.1 g Sugar 3.4 g

Protein 17.9 g Cholesterol 52 mg

Creamy Chicken Penne

Preparation Time: 10 minutes

Cooking Time: 6 hours

Servings: 6

Ingredients:

3 chicken breasts, boneless & skinless

1 lb penne pasta, cooked

2 cups cheddar cheese, shredded

1 cup sour cream

1/2 onion, diced

1 1/2 cups mushrooms, sliced

1/2 tsp dried thyme

1/2 cup chicken broth

21 oz can cream of chicken soup

Pepper

Salt

Directions:

Add chicken, soup, onions, mushrooms, thyme, pepper, and broth into the cooking pot and stir well.

Cover instant pot aura with lid. Select slow cook mode and cook on LOW for 6 hours. Remove chicken from pot and shred using a fork, return shredded chicken to the pot and stir well.

Stir in cheddar cheese, penne, and sour cream.

Serve and enjoy.

Nutrition:

Calories 690 Fat 33.6 g Carbohydrates 52.2 g

Sugar 1.6 g Protein 43.7 g Cholesterol 185 mg

Tasty Chicken Fajita Pasta

Preparation Time: 10 minutes
Cooking Time: 6 hours
Servings: 6
Ingredients:
2 chicken breasts, skinless & boneless
2 cups cheddar cheese, shredded
16 oz penne pasta, cooked
2 cups chicken broth
10 oz can tomato, diced
2 tsp garlic, minced
1 bell peppers, diced
1/2 onion, diced
2 tbsp taco seasoning

Directions:
Add all ingredients except cheese and pasta into the cooking pot and stir well.
Cover instant pot aura with lid.
Select slow cook mode and cook on LOW for 6 hours.

Stir in cheese and pasta.

Serve and enjoy.

Nutrition:

Calories 620

Fat 25.2 g

Carbohydrates 56.2 g

Sugar 3.4 g

Protein 41.3 g

Cholesterol 157 mg

Moist & Juicy Chicken Breast

Preparation Time: 10 minutes

Cooking Time: 3 hours

Servings: 4

Ingredients:

4 chicken breasts, skinless and boneless

1/8 tsp paprika

1 tbsp butter

1/4 cup chicken broth

1/8 tsp onion powder

1/4 tsp garlic powder

1/2 tsp dried parsley

1/8 tsp pepper

1/2 tsp salt

Directions:

In a small bowl, mix together paprika, onion powder, garlic powder, parsley, pepper, and salt.

Rub chicken breasts with a spice mixture from both the sides.

Add broth and butter to the cooking pot and stir to combine.

Add chicken to the cooking pot.

Cover instant pot aura with lid.

Select slow cook mode and cook on LOW for 3 hours.

Serve and enjoy.

Nutrition:

Calories 307 Fat 13.8 g Carbohydrates 0.4 g

Sugar 0.1 g Protein 42.6 g Cholesterol 138 mg

Asian Chicken

Preparation Time: 10 minutes

Cooking Time: 6 hours

Servings: 4

Ingredients:

4 chicken breasts, skinless and boneless

1/2 cup of soy sauce

1 tbsp ginger, minced

3 garlic cloves, chopped

1 onion, chopped

3 tbsp sesame seeds

1/3 cup rice vinegar

1/3 cup honey

Directions:

Add chicken into the cooking pot.

Add ginger, garlic, and onion on top of the chicken.

Add vinegar, honey, and soy sauce to the cooking pot.

Season with pepper and salt.

Cover instant pot aura with lid.

Select slow cook mode and cook on LOW for 6 hours.

Shred chicken using a fork and stir well.

Serve and enjoy.

Nutrition:

Calories 451 Fat 14.3 g Carbohydrates 31.6 g Sugar 25 g Protein 46.1 g Cholesterol 130 mg

Flavorful Chicken Casserole

Preparation Time: 10 minutes

Cooking Time: 8 hours

Servings: 6

Ingredients:

4 chicken breasts, boneless & skinless

1 1/2 cups chicken stock

10.5 oz can cream of chicken soup

15 oz can corn kernels, drained

2 cups cheddar cheese, shredded

1 cup cooked rice

1 onion, chopped

Directions:

Add chicken into the cooking pot.

Add chopped onion over chicken.

In a bowl, stir together stock and soup and pour over the chicken.

Cover instant pot aura with lid.

Select slow cook mode and cook on LOW for 8 hours.

Remove chicken from cooking pot and shred using a fork.

Return shredded chicken to the cooking pot along with corn, cheese, and rice. Stir well.

Serve and enjoy.

Nutrition:

Calories 561 Fat 23.6 g Carbohydrates 43.9 g

Sugar 3.6 g Protein 43.2 g Cholesterol 130 mg

Chicken Orzo

Preparation Time: 10 minutes
Cooking Time: 4 hours 30 minutes
Servings: 4
Ingredients:
1 lb chicken breasts, skinless and boneless, cut in half
3/4 cup whole wheat orzo
1 tsp Italian herbs
1 lemon juice
2 tbsp green onion, chopped
1/3 cup olives
1 lemon zest, grated
1 onion, sliced
1 cup chicken stock
1/2 cup bell pepper, diced
2 tomatoes, chopped

Directions:
Add all ingredients except olives and orzo into the cooking pot and stir well.

Cover instant pot aura with lid.

Select slow cook mode and cook on LOW for 4 hours.

Stir in olives and orzo and cook for 30 minutes more.

Serve and enjoy.

Nutrition:

Calories 333 Fat 10.6 g Carbohydrates 22.3 g

Sugar 4.8 g Protein 36.4 g

Cholesterol 101 mg

Garlic Herb Roasted Pepper Chicken

Preparation Time: 10 minutes

Cooking Time: 4 hours

Servings: 6

Ingredients:

2 lbs chicken thighs, skinless and boneless

1 cup roasted red peppers, chopped

1/2 cup chicken stock

1 cup olives

1 tsp rosemary

1 tsp dried thyme

1 tsp oregano

1 tbsp capers

3 garlic cloves, minced

1 onion, sliced

1 tbsp olive oil

Pepper

Salt

Directions:

Add all ingredients into the cooking pot and stir well.

Cover instant pot aura with lid.

Select slow cook mode and cook on LOW for 4 hours.

Stir well and serve.

Nutrition:

Calories 354 Fat 16.1 g Carbohydrates 6 g

Sugar 2.2 g Protein 44.7 g Cholesterol 135 mg

Slow Cook Turkey Breast

Preparation Time: 10 minutes
Cooking Time: 4 hours 30 minutes
Servings: 6
Ingredients:
4 lbs turkey breast
1/2 fresh lemon juice
1/2 cup sun-dried tomatoes, chopped
1/2 cup olives, chopped
3 tbsp flour
3/4 cup chicken stock
4 garlic cloves, chopped
1 tsp dried oregano
1 onion, chopped
1/4 tsp pepper
1/2 tsp salt
Directions:

Add turkey breast, garlic, oregano, lemon juice, sun-dried tomatoes, olives, onion, pepper, and salt to the cooking pot.

Pour half stock over turkey.

Cover instant pot aura with lid.

Select slow cook mode and cook on LOW for 4 hours.

Whisk together remaining stock and flour and add into the cooking pot and stir well, cover, and cook on LOW for 30 minutes more.

Serve and enjoy.

Nutrition:

Calories 358 Fat 6.5 g Carbohydrates 19.8 g

Sugar 12 g Protein 52.7 g Cholesterol 130 mg

Simple Chicken & Mushrooms

Preparation Time: 10 minutes

Cooking Time: 6 hours

Servings: 2

Ingredients:

2 chicken breasts, skinless and boneless

1 cup mushrooms, sliced

1/2 tsp thyme, dried

1 onion, sliced

1 cup chicken stock

Pepper

Salt

Directions:

Add all ingredients into the cooking pot and stir well.

Cover instant pot aura with lid.

Select slow cook mode and cook on LOW for 6 hours.

Stir well and serve. Nutrition:

Calories 313 Fat 11.3 g Carbohydrates 6.9 g

Lemon Herb Chicken

Preparation Time: 10 minutes

Cooking Time: 4 hours

Servings: 4

Ingredients:

20 oz chicken breasts, skinless, boneless, and cut into pieces

3/4 cup chicken broth

1/2 tsp dried oregano

1 tsp dried parsley

2 tbsp olive oil

2 tbsp butter

1/2 cup fresh lemon juice

1/8 tsp dried thyme

1/4 tsp dried basil

3 tbsp rice flour

1 tsp salt

Directions:

In a bowl, toss chicken with rice flour.

Add butter and olive oil in a cooking pot and set instant pot aura on saute mode.

Add chicken to the cooking pot and cook until brown.

Add remaining ingredients on top of the chicken.

Cover instant pot aura with lid.

Select slow cook mode and cook on LOW for 4 hours.

Serve and enjoy.

Nutrition:

Calories 423 Fat 23.9 g

Carbohydrates 6.9 g Sugar 0.8 g

Protein 42.7 g

Cholesterol 141 mg

Creamy Chicken Curry

Preparation Time: 10 minutes

Cooking Time: 6 hours

Servings: 6

Ingredients:

1 1/2 lbs chicken thighs, boneless

1/2 cup chicken broth

3 potatoes, peeled and cut into 1-inch pieces

15 oz can coconut milk

2 tbsp brown sugar

1/2 tsp red pepper, crushed

1/2 tsp coriander, crushed

2 tbsp curry powder

3 tbsp fresh ginger, chopped

1/2 tsp black pepper

1 tsp kosher salt

Directions:

Add all ingredients into the cooking pot and stir well.

Cover instant pot aura with lid.

Select slow cook mode and cook on LOW for 6 hours.

Stir well and serve.

Nutrition:

Calories 463 Fat 24.2 g

Carbohydrates 25.7 g Sugar 4.8 g

Protein 37.1 g Cholesterol 101 mg

Taco Chicken

Preparation Time: 10 minutes
Cooking Time: 6 hours
Servings: 8
Ingredients:
1 lb chicken breasts, skinless and boneless
2 tbsp taco seasoning
1 cup chicken broth
Directions:
Add all ingredients into the cooking pot and stir well.
Cover instant pot aura with lid. Select slow cook mode and cook on LOW for 6 hours.
Remove chicken from pot and shred using a fork, return shredded chicken to the pot. Stir well and serve.
Nutrition:
Calories 118 Fat 4.7 g Carbohydrates 0.5 g
Sugar 0.1 g Protein 17.3 g Cholesterol 51 mg

Butter Chicken

Preparation Time: 10 minutes

Cooking Time: 5 hours

Servings: 5

Ingredients:

1 lb chicken thighs, boneless and skinless

1 lb chicken breasts, boneless and skinless

1 1/2 tbsp ginger paste

1 tbsp garam masala

1 tbsp curry powder

1/3 cup heavy whipping cream

1 1/2 tbsp butter - 1/4 cup tomato paste

1/2 cup chicken broth

3/4 tsp kosher salt

Directions:

Cut chicken into the cooking pot. pour remaining ingredients except whipping cream over chicken and stir well. Cover instant pot aura with lid. Select slow cook mode and cook on LOW for 5 hours. Stir in cream and serve.

Nutrition:

Calories 427 Fat 20.3 g Carbohydrates 4.7 g

Spicy Chili Chicken

Preparation Time: 10 minutes

Cooking Time: 6 hours

Servings: 5

Ingredients:

1 lb chicken breasts, skinless and boneless

1 jalapeno pepper, chopped

1 poblano pepper, chopped

12 oz can green chilies

1/2 cup dried chives

1/2 tsp paprika

1/2 tsp dried sage

1/2 tsp cumin

1 tsp dried oregano

14 oz can tomato, diced

2 cups of water

1 tsp sea salt

Directions:

Add all ingredients into the cooking pot and stir well.

Cover instant pot aura with lid.

Select slow cook mode and cook on LOW for 6 hours.

Remove chicken from pot and shred using a fork, return shredded chicken to the pot.

Stir well and serve.

Nutrition:

Calories 212 Fat 7.1 g Carbohydrates 8.9 g

Sugar 3.4 g Protein 27.9 g

Cholesterol 81 mg

Pesto Chicken

Preparation Time: 10 minutes

Cooking Time: 7 hours

Servings: 2

Ingredients:

2 chicken breasts, skinless and boneless

2 cups cherry tomatoes, halved

2 tbsp basil pesto

2 cups zucchini, chopped

2 cups green beans, chopped

Directions:

Add all ingredients into the cooking pot and stir well. Cover instant pot aura with lid. Select slow cook mode and cook on LOW for 7 hours. Stir well and serve.

Nutrition:

Calories 26 Fat 0.8 g Carbohydrates 1.3 g

Sugar 0.6 g Protein 3.4 g Cholesterol 9 mg

Rosemary Turkey Breast

Preparation Time: 10 minutes
Cooking Time: 4 hours
Servings: 12
Ingredients:
6 lbs turkey breast, bone-in

4 fresh rosemary sprigs

1/2 cup water

Pepper

Salt

Directions:
Add all ingredients into the cooking pot and stir well. Cover instant pot aura with lid.

Select slow cook mode and cook on LOW for 4 hours.

Serve and enjoy.

Nutrition:
Calories 237 Fat 3.8 g Carbohydrates 9.8 g

Sugar 8 g Protein 38.7 g Cholesterol 98 mg

Garlic Olive Chicken

Preparation Time: 10 minutes
Cooking Time: 6 hours
Servings: 4
Ingredients:
2 1/2 lbs chicken legs

1 tbsp capers

5 garlic cloves, smashed

3 tbsp red wine vinegar

1 1/2 tsp dried oregano

1/3 cup white wine

1/4 cup fresh parsley, chopped

1/3 cup olives, pitted

1/2 cup prunes

Pepper

Salt

Directions:
Add all ingredients into the cooking pot and stir well.

Cover instant pot aura with lid. Select slow cook mode and cook on LOW for 4 hours.

Serve and enjoy.

Nutrition:

Calories 630 Fat 22.4 g Carbohydrates 16.9 g

Sugar 8.4 g Protein 83 g Cholesterol 252 mg

Delicious Chickpea Chicken

Preparation Time: 10 minutes
Cooking Time: 4 hours
Servings: 4
Ingredients:
2 lbs chicken thighs

1 tsp paprika

1 tbsp lemon juice

2 tbsp olive oil

1 tsp garlic, minced

3 cups grape tomatoes, sliced

14 oz can chickpeas, drained and rinsed

1 tsp chili powder

1 tsp curry powder

1 tsp cumin

1 tsp oregano

1 tsp coriander

1 lemon, sliced

1 tsp salt

Directions:

Add all ingredients into the cooking pot and stir well. Cover instant pot aura with lid. Select slow cook mode and cook on LOW for 4 hours. Serve and enjoy.

Nutrition:

Calories 648 Fat 25.7 g Carbohydrates 30.8 g Sugar 4.1 g Protein 72.3 g Cholesterol 202 mg

Chicken Kale Soup

Preparation Time: 15 minutes
Cooking Time: 6 hours
Servings: 6
Ingredients:

1 tablespoon olive oil

14 ounces chicken broth

0.5 cups olive oil

5 ounces kale

Salt to taste

2 pounds of chicken

0.33 cups onion

32 ounces chicken stock

0.25 cups lemon juice

Directions:

Cook the chicken until it achieves approximately 165F. Do this in a pan.

Shred and put it into the cooker.

Process the onion, broth, and oil and put it into the cooker.

Add other ingredients and mix.

Low cook for 6 hours. Serve.

Nutrition:

Calories 261 Fat 21 g

Protein 14 g Carbs 2 g

Creamy Italian Chicken

Preparation Time: 15 minutes

Cooking Time: 6 hours

Servings: 8

Ingredients:

2 pounds of chicken

10.5 ounces chicken soup, cream and canned

1 teaspoon garlic powder

0.25 cups onion

2 tablespoons dressing mix, Italian

8 ounces cream cheese

Directions:

Cube the chicken. Place it in the cooker.

Dice and add onions. Stir in cream cheese: mix garlic, soup, and dressing mix.

Pour into the cooker. Low cook for 6 hours.

Nutrition:

Calories 255 Fat 14 g Protein 23 g Carbs 7 g

Chicken and Vegetables

Preparation Time: 15 minutes

Cooking Time: 8 hours

Servings: 8

Ingredients:

2 pounds chicken that does not contain any skin or bones

2 cups green beans

1 cup chicken broth

2 teaspoons herb blend

2 cups carrots

2 onions

4 teaspoons Worcestershire sauce

Pepper and salt

Directions:

Prepare and chop the vegetables. Put the chicken in the cooker. Add the vegetables. Pour the broth and Worcestershire sauce. Low cook for 8 hours.

Nutrition:

Chicken Gyros

Preparation Time: 15 minutes
Cooking Time: 8 hours
Servings: 8
Ingredients:

0.5 an onion

2 pounds ground chicken

0.5 cups breadcrumbs, low-carb

1 teaspoon thyme

0.25 teaspoons nutmeg

1 tablespoon olive oil

3 garlic cloves

2 eggs

1 lemon

0.25 teaspoons cinnamon

12 pita bread

Toppings:

Tomato

Greek yogurt, plain

Cucumber

Lemon

Directions:

Process the garlic and onion. Mix the above with the eggs, lemon, cinnamon, salt, chicken, breadcrumbs, thyme, and nutmeg.

Roll into a ball. Put in a cooker—drizzle olive oil.

Low cook for 8 hours. Once finished, put on pita and apply toppings.

Nutrition:

Calories 248 Fat 13 g Protein 23 g Carbs 10 g

Crockpot Creamy Salsa Chicken

Preparation Time: 15 minutes

Cooking Time: 4 hours

Servings: 4

Ingredients:

1/2 jar salsa

1/2 can of cream mushroom soup

3 large boneless chicken breasts

Directions:

Lay and settle the chicken breasts inside the slow cooker.

Combine in the salsa plus the mushroom soup. Set it on top of the chicken breasts.

Cook on low within 4 hours, stirring occasionally, and shred once cooked, then serve.

Nutrition:

Calories 254.6 Protein 40.8g Carbs 5.3g Fat 6.6g

Pizza Casserole

Preparation Time: 15 minutes

Cooking Time: 4 hours

Servings: 3

Ingredients:

2 chicken breasts without bones

2 garlic cloves

1 teaspoon seasoning, Italian

Dash pepper

8 ounces tomato sauce

1 bay leaf

0.25 teaspoons salt

0.5 cups mozzarella

Directions:

Put the chicken in the cooker. Add other ingredients, except cheese.

Low cook for 4 hours. After cooking, top with cheese.

Nutrition:

Calories 228 Fat 9 g Protein 31 g Carbs 5 g

Moist and Spicy Pulled Chicken Breast

Preparation Time: 15 minutes

Cooking Time: 6 hours

Servings: 8

Ingredients:

1 teaspoon dry oregano

1 teaspoon dry thyme

1 teaspoon dried rosemary

1 teaspoon garlic powder

1 teaspoon sweet paprika

½ teaspoon chili powder

Salt and pepper to taste

4 tablespoons butter

5.5 pounds of chicken breasts

1 ½ cups ready-made tomato salsa

2 Tablespoons of olive oil

Directions:

Mix dry seasoning, sprinkle half on the bottom of crockpot. Place the chicken breasts over it, sprinkle the rest of the spices.

Pour the salsa over the chicken. Cover, cook on low for 6 hours.

Nutrition:

Calories: 42 Carbs: 1g Fat: 1g Protein: 9g

Whole Roasted Chicken

Preparation Time: 15 minutes

Cooking Time: 8 hours

Servings: 6

Ingredients:

1 whole chicken (approximately 5.5 pounds)

4 garlic cloves

6 small onions

1 Tablespoon olive oil, for rubbing

2 teaspoons salt

2 teaspoons sweet paprika

1 teaspoon Cayenne pepper

1 teaspoon onion powder

1 teaspoon ground thyme

2 teaspoons fresh ground black pepper

4 Tablespoons butter, cut into cubes

Directions:

Mix all dry ingredients well.

Stuff the chicken belly with garlic and onions.

On the bottom of the crockpot, place four balls of aluminum foil.

Set the chicken on top of the balls. Rub it generously with olive oil.

Cover the chicken with seasoning, drop in butter pieces. Cover, cook on low for 8 hours.

Nutrition:

Calories: 120 Carbs: 1g Fat: 6g Protein: 17g

Simple Chicken Chili

Preparation Time: 15 minutes

Cooking Time: 6 hours

Servings: 8

Ingredients:

1 Tablespoon butter

1 red onion, sliced

1 bell pepper, sliced

2 garlic cloves, minced

3 pounds boneless chicken thighs

8 slices bacon, chopped

1 teaspoon chili powder

Salt and pepper to taste

1 cup chicken broth

¼ cup of coconut milk

3 Tablespoons tomato paste

Directions:

Add all ingredients to the crockpot, starting with the butter.

Cover, cook on low for 6 hours.

Strip the chicken using a fork in the crockpot. Serve.

Nutrition:

Calories: 210

Carbs: 32g

Fat: 4g

Protein: 14g

Chicken in Salsa Verde

Preparation Time: 15 minutes
Cooking Time: 6 hours
Servings: 4

Ingredients:

2.2 pounds of chicken breasts

3 bunches parsley, chopped

¾ cup olive oil

¼ cup capers, drained and chopped

3 anchovy fillets

1 lemon, juice, and zest

2 garlic cloves, minced

1 teaspoon salt

1 teaspoon fresh ground black pepper

Directions:

Place the chicken breasts in the crockpot.

Blend the rest of the fixing in a blender, then pour over the chicken.

Cover, cook on low for 6 hours. Shred with a fork and serve.

Nutrition:

Calories: 145 Carbs: 5g Fat: 2g Protein: 26g

Egg Casserole with Italian Cheeses, Sun-Dried Tomatoes, and Herbs

Preparation Time: 5 minutes

Cooking Time: 4 hours

Servings: 8

Ingredients:

10 eggs

2 tablespoons milk

3 tablespoons sun-dried tomatoes, chopped

2 tablespoons onion, minced

2 tablespoons basil, chopped

1 tablespoon thyme leaves

Salt and pepper to taste

1 cup mixed Italian cheeses, grated

Directions:

Mix all items in a bowl. Put it inside your slow cooker, and set to cook on high for 2 hours or low for 3 hours.

Egg and Cheese Casserole with Chayote Squash

Preparation Time: 5 minutes
Cooking Time: 4 hours
Servings: 4
Ingredients:

1 teaspoon olive oil

1 red onion, diced

2 small chayote squash, grated

½ small red bell pepper, diced

10 large eggs, beaten

¼ cup low-fat cottage cheese

2 tablespoons milk

½ teaspoon ground cumin

2 cups grated cheesed

Salt and pepper to taste

Directions:

Combine all fixings in a mixing bowl. Pour into the slow cooker.

Cook on high within 3 hours or on low for 4 hours.

Nutrition:

Calories: 209 Carbohydrates: 6.3g

Protein: 35.2g Fat: 33.6g

Sugar: 1.5g Sodium: 362mg Fiber: 3.2g

Scrambled Eggs with Smoked Salmon

Preparation Time: 15 minutes
Cooking Time: 2 hours
Servings: 6
Ingredients:

smoked salmon ¼ lb.

eggs12 pcs fresh

heavy cream½ cup

almond flour¼ cup

Salt and black pepper at will

Butter2 tablespoons

fresh chives at will

Directions:

Cut the slices of salmon. Set aside for garnish. Chop the rest of the salmon into small pieces.

Take a medium bowl, whisk the eggs and cream together. Add half of the chopped chives, season eggs with salt and pepper. Add flour.

Dissolve the butter over medium heat, then pour into the mixture. Grease the Slow Cooker with oil or cooking spray. Add salmon pieces to the mixture, pour it into the Slow Cooker. Set to cook on low within 2 hours.

Garnish the dish with remaining salmon, chives. Serve warm and enjoy!

Nutrition:

Calories: 263

Carbs: 0g

Fat: 0g

Protein: 0g

PORK & LAMB

Mouth-Watering Minced Pork Zucchini Lasagna

Preparation Time: 15 minutes

Cooking Time: 8 hours

Servings: 4

Ingredients:

4 medium zucchinis

1 diced small onion

1 minced clove of garlic

2 cups of minced lean ground pork

2 cans of Italian diced tomatoes

2 tablespoons of olive oil

2 cups of shredded Mozzarella cheese

1 large egg

1 tablespoon of dried basil

Salt and pepper

2 tablespoons of butter

Directions:

Slice the zucchini lengthwise into 6 slices. Heat-up the olive oil in a saucepan, then sauté the garlic and onions for 5 minutes.

Put the minced meat, cook for a further 5 minutes, put the tomatoes, and cook for an additional 5 minutes. Add the seasoning and mix thoroughly.

Mix the egg plus cheese in a small bowl, and whisk. Grease the crockpot using the butter, and then begin to layer the lasagna. First, layer with the zucchini slices, add the meat mixture, then top with the cheese. Repeat and finish with the cheese—Cook for 8 hours on low.

Nutrition:

Carbs: 10 g

Protein: 23 g

Fat: 30 g

Calories: 398

Beautiful BBQ Ribs

Preparation Time: 15 minutes

Cooking Time: 8 hours

Servings: 4

Ingredients:

3 pounds of pork ribs

1 tablespoon of olive oil

1 can of tomato paste, 28 ounces

½ cup of hot water

½ cup of vinegar

6 tablespoons of Worcestershire sauce

4 tablespoons of dry mustard

1 tablespoon of chili powder

1 teaspoon of ground cumin

1 teaspoon of powdered sweetener of your choice

Salt and pepper

Directions:

Heat the olive oil in a large frying pan and brown the ribs, then put in the crockpot.

Combine the remainder of the fixing in a small bowl, whisk thoroughly and pour over the ribs—Cook for 8 hours on low.

Nutrition:

Carbs: 14 g Protein: 38 g Fat: 28 g Calories: 410

Gorgeous Coconut Turmeric Pork Curry

Preparation Time: 15 minutes

Cooking Time: 8 hours

Servings: 4

Ingredients:

2.2 pounds of cubed pork shoulder

1 tablespoon of coconut oil

1 tablespoon of olive oil

1 diced yellow onion

2 cloves of minced garlic

2 tablespoons of tomato paste

1 can of coconut milk, 12 ounces

1 cup of water

½ cup of white wine

1 teaspoon of turmeric

1 teaspoon of ginger powder

1 teaspoon of curry powder

½ teaspoon of paprika

Salt and pepper

Directions:

Heat-up 1 tablespoon of olive oil in a saucepan and sauté the garlic and onions for 3 minutes.

Add the pork and brown it, and then add the tomato paste.

Mix the remaining ingredients in the crockpot and then add the pork.

Cook for 8 hours on low. Divide onto plates and serve

Nutrition:

Carbs: 7 g Protein: 30 g Fat: 31 g Calories: 425

Kalua Pork

Preparation Time: 15 minutes

Cooking Time: 8 hours

Servings: 8

Ingredients:

4 lbs. pork shoulder roast

1 tbsp liquid smoke

2 tsp sea salt

Directions:

Place pork roast into the slow cooker. Pour liquid smoke and sea salt all over the pork roast.

Cook within 8 hours, low. Shred the meat, then serve.

Nutrition:

Calories 582 Fat 46.2 g Carbohydrates 0 g

Sugar 0 g Protein 38.1 g

Cholesterol 161 mg Fiber 0 g

Tasty Cuban Mojo Pork

Preparation Time: 15 minutes

Cooking Time: 8 hours

Servings: 6

Ingredients:

2 lbs. pork shoulder, boneless and cut into 2 pieces

2 bay leaves

1/2 tsp paprika

1/2 tsp cumin

1 1/2 tsp dried oregano

1/2 tsp pepper

3 garlic cloves, minced

1 jalapeno pepper, halved

1 small onion, chopped

1 lime zest

1/4 cup lime juice

1/2 cup orange juice

1/4 cup vinegar

3/4 cup chicken broth

1 tsp salt

Directions:

Place pork roast into the slow cooker. Add remaining ingredients into the slow cooker.

Cook within 8 hours, low setting. Discard bay leaves and shred the meat using a fork. Serve and enjoy.

Nutrition:

Calories 468 Fat 32.7 g Carbohydrates 4.6 g

Sugar 2.5 g Protein 36.3 g Cholesterol 136 mg

Fiber 0.7 g Net carbs 4.6 g

Slow Cooker Pork Loin

Preparation Time: 15 minutes
Cooking Time: 6 hours
Servings: 4
Ingredients:

1/4 cup orange juice

1/2 tbsp curry powder

1/2 tsp chicken bouillon granules

1/4 tsp ground ginger

1/8 tsp ground cinnamon

1/4 tsp salt

1/2 onion, diced

1/2 garlic, diced

1/8 cup raisins

1/8 cup flaked coconut

1 tbsp cold water

2 pounds boneless pork loin, diced

1 tbsp arrowroot powder

Directions:

Mix the salt, cinnamon, chicken bouillon, curry powder, and orange in the slow cooker's bottom.

Mix in the coconut, raisins, garlic, onion, and apple, then place the pork cubes into the mixture.

Put the potato starch into water, mix until it dissolved. Then put all inside the slow cooker.

Cook on low within 5 to 6 hours.

Nutrition:

Calories 174 Fat 6g Carbs 8g Protein 22g

Green Chili Pork

Preparation Time: 15 minutes
Cooking Time: 8 hours
Servings: 8
Ingredients:

3 lbs. boneless pork, cubed

2 garlic cloves, minced

16 oz stewed tomatoes

4 oz green chilies, chopped

1 cup chicken broth

1 tsp oregano

1 tsp cumin

1 small onion, chopped

1 tbsp olive oil

Pepper

Salt

Directions:

Heat-up the olive oil in a pan medium-high heat. Brown the pork in hot oil. Transfer pork into the slow cooker.

Add remaining ingredients and stir well—Cook within 8 hours, low. Serve and enjoy.

Nutrition:

Calories 284

Fat 8.1 g

Carbohydrates 4.6 g

Sugar 2.5 g

Protein 45.9 g

Cholesterol 124 mg

Fiber 1 g

Net carbs 3.6 g

Thai Curried Pork

Preparation Time: 15 minutes
Cooking Time: 8 hours
Servings: 6
Ingredients:

4 pork chops, boneless

1/2 cup chicken broth

1 tsp red pepper flakes

2 tsp cardamom

2 tsp cumin

1 tbsp curry powder

1 tbsp turmeric

8 oz baby carrots, peeled and chopped

1 tbsp fresh ginger, grated

4 garlic cloves, minced

1 small onion, chopped

Pepper

Sea salt

Directions:

Spray slow cooker from inside with cooking spray. Put all the items into the slow cooker, and stir well.

Cook within 8 hours, low. Shred the pork chops using a fork. Serve and enjoy.

Nutrition:

Calories 211 Fat 14 g

Carbohydrates 7.9 g

Sugar 2.5 g Protein 13.4 g

Cholesterol 46 mg

Fiber 2.4 g

Net carbs 5.5 g

Chinese 5-Spice Pork Ribs

Preparation Time: 15 minutes
Cooking Time: 8 hours
Servings: 6
Ingredients:

3 lbs. (1.36kg) baby back pork ribs

Salt and pepper to taste

2 teaspoons Chinese five-spice powder

3/4 teaspoon coarse garlic powder

1 fresh jalapeño, cut into rings

2 tablespoons rice vinegar

2 tablespoons coconut aminos (or soy sauce)

1 tablespoon tomato paste

Directions:

Start by cutting the ribs in the pieces so they'll fit into the slow cooker. Massage with salt and pepper.

Mix the Chinese 5-spice mixture and garlic and massage into the meat in a small bowl.

Place the jalapeño rings into the bottom of your slow cooker, followed by the rice vinegar, the coconut aminos, and the tomato paste and stir it all together until combined.

Add the ribs but stand them up, pop the lid back on and cook for 6-8 hours on high.

Cook until the ribs almost fall apart.

Nutrition:

Calories: 164 Carbs: 6g Fat: 7g Protein: 19g

Pork Stew with Oyster Mushrooms

Preparation Time: 15 minutes
Cooking Time: 8 hours
Servings: 4
Ingredients:

2 tablespoons butter or lard

1 medium onion, chopped

1 clove garlic, chopped

2lbs (900g) pork loin, cut into 1" cubes and patted dry

½ teaspoon salt

½ teaspoon freshly cracked black pepper

2 tablespoons dried oregano

2 tablespoons dried mustard

½ teaspoon ground nutmeg

1½ cups (355ml) bone broth or stock

2 tablespoons white wine vinegar

2 lbs. (900g) oyster mushrooms

¼ cup (60ml) full-fat coconut milk

¼ cup (60ml) ghee

3 tablespoons capers

Directions:

Turn your slow cooker onto a high heat and melt the butter or lard. Add the meat and cook well until brown on both sides. Remove the meat but keep the juices at the bottom. Add some more fat and add the onions and garlic and cook for around 5 minutes until soft.

Add the oregano, mustard, nutmeg, broth, and vinegar and stir well to combine. Return the meat into the slow cooker, then cover with the lid and cook for 6 hours on low.

Remove the lid, throw in the mushrooms and an extra cup of water and cook for a further 1-2 hours.

Whisk in the coconut milk, ghee, and capers, then serve and enjoy!

Nutrition:

Calories: 190 Carbs: 0g Fat: 10g Protein: 23g

Paprika Pork Tenderloin

Preparation Time: 15 minutes
Cooking Time: 4 hours & 20 minutes
Servings: 4
Ingredients:

1 ½ lb. lean pork tenderloin

½ teaspoon salt

2 tablespoons paprika, smoked

1 cup chicken broth

1 tablespoon oregano

½ cup of salsa

Black pepper

Directions:

Pour chicken stock in a small mixing bowl.

Add salsa, pepper, paprika, salt, and oregano. Mix well.

Remove the fat from the pork before placing it in the slow cooker. Add the liquid mixture.

Cook within 4 hours on high.

Shred the pork, then cook for another 20 minutes without cover.

Nutrition:

Calories: 160 Carbs: 2g

Fat: 8g

Protein: 22g

Pork Carnitas

Preparation Time: 15 minutes
Cooking Time: 8 hours
Servings: 16
Ingredients:
8 lb. Boston pork butt

1 cup of water

2 tablespoons butter

2 tablespoons chili powder

4 tablespoons garlic, minced

1 large onion, sliced thin

1 tablespoon pepper

2 tablespoons cumin

1 tablespoon salt

2 tablespoons thyme

Directions:
Grease the slow cooker using butter. Distribute onion and garlic evenly in the bottom of the slow cooker.

Remove the fat from the meat and lightly slice the top with a crisscross pattern. Mix the spices in a bowl, then coat the meat with it.

Put meat in the slow cooker with water—Cook for about 8 hours, high.

Nutrition:

Calories: 200 Carbs: 0g Fat: 14g Protein: 20g

Lemongrass Coconut Pulled Pork

Preparation Time: 15 minutes
Cooking Time: 8 hours
Servings: 8
Ingredients:

3 lb. butt roast or pork loin

½ cup of coconut milk

2-inch ginger, sliced

3 tablespoons lemongrass, minced

1 onion, sliced

3 cloves garlic, minced

1 teaspoon ground pepper

2 teaspoons kosher salt

1 tablespoon apple cider vinegar

3 tablespoons olive oil

Directions:

Remove fat from the roast and cut a crisscross pattern into it. Distribute onion and ginger slices evenly at the bottom of a slow cooker.

Mix olive oil, pepper, salt, apple cider vinegar, lemongrass, and garlic in a bowl until a loose paste is formed. Coat the pork with the mixture and put it in the slow cooker.

Cover and leave it overnight. Once done, pour coconut milk into the slow cooker and set it on low—Cook for 8 hours. Shred the meat using forks.

Nutrition:

Calories: 120 Carbs: 0g Fat: 3g Protein: 23g

Pork Loin Roast with Onion Gravy

Preparation Time: 15 minutes
Cooking Time: 6 hours
Servings: 6
Ingredients:

4 lb. pork loin roast

2 tablespoons coconut aminos

1 tablespoon of sea salt

¼ cup of water

2 teaspoon black pepper

2 medium onions, sliced

2 cloves garlic, minced

Directions:

Put pepper, salt, and garlic in a bowl and mix well. Use it to coat all sides of the roast.

Distribute onion slices in the slow cooker. Pour in coconut aminos and water.

Put the roast in the slow cooker.

Cook within 4-6 hours, low.

Transfer the cooking juices and onions into a blender.

Process until smooth.

Pour mixture over pork roast.

Nutrition:

Calories: 190 Carbs: 5g Fat: 10g Protein: 18g

Lime Pork Chops

Preparation Time: 15 minutes
Cooking Time: 4 hours
Servings: 8
Ingredients:

3.32 lb. pork sirloin

¾ teaspoon black pepper

3 tablespoons butter

½ ground cumin

¾ teaspoon salt

½ cup of salsa

¾ teaspoon garlic powder

5 tablespoons lime juice

Directions:

Mix all of the flavorings in a small bowl. Cover the meat all over with the flavoring mixture.

Using a pan, sear the meat in butter over medium-high heat until brown on both sides.

Combine lime juice and salsa in a separate bowl. Mix well.

Put the pork chops inside the slow cooker and pour the salsa mixture on top. Cook within 3-4 hours, low.

Nutrition:

Calories: 170 Carbs: 8g Fat: 6g Protein: 18g

Chili Pulled Pork

Preparation Time: 15 minutes
Cooking Time: 10 hours
Servings: 10
Ingredients:

4 1/2 lb. (2kg) pork butt / shoulder

2 tablespoons chili powder

1 tablespoon salt

1 ½ teaspoon ground cumin

½ teaspoon ground oregano

¼ teaspoon crushed red pepper flakes

Pinch ground cloves

½ cup (120ml) stock or bone broth

1 bay leaf

Directions:

Start by grabbing a bowl and throwing in the chili, salt, cumin, oregano, red pepper flakes, and a pinch of cloves then stir well to combine. Lay the pork out on a clean plate, remove the skin if applicable, then rub the spice mixture into the pork. Put into the fridge within 1-2 hours.

When you're ready to cook, pop the pork in the bottom of the slow cooker, add the bay leaf and the stock or broth, replace the lid and switch on. Cook on low for 8-10 hours (or overnight) until tender.

Remove the lid, lift the pork from the slow cooker, and place onto a cutting board then shred with two forks. Serve and enjoy!

Nutrition:

Calories: 210 Carbs: 0g Fat: 15g Protein: 0g

Ranch Pork Chops

Preparation Time: 15 minutes

Cooking Time: 6 hours

Servings: 8

Ingredients:

3 lbs. pork chops

1 tsp garlic powder

1 oz ranch dressing mix

1 oz onion soup mix

22.5 oz cream of mushroom soup

1/2 tsp black pepper

Directions:

Spray slow cooker form inside with cooking spray. Put all listed items into the slow cooker, then mix well.

Cook within 6 hours on low. Serve and enjoy.

Nutrition:

Calories 591 Fat 44.6 g Carbohydrates 5.4 g

Sugar 0.9 g Protein 39.2 g Cholesterol 146 mg

Fiber 0.3 g Net carbs 5.1 g

Delicious Coconut Pork

Preparation Time: 15 minutes
Cooking Time: 8 hours
Servings: 6
Ingredients:

3 lbs. pork shoulder, boneless and cut into chunks

1/2 cup fresh cilantro, chopped

1 1/2 cups coconut water

1/4 cup fish sauce

2 tbsp olive oil

5 scallions, chopped

Directions:

Heat-up olive oil in a pan over medium heat. Brown the meat in hot oil. Transfer meat into the slow cooker.

Add the rest of the items into the slow cooker and mix well. Cook on low within 8 hours. Serve and enjoy.

Nutrition:

Calories 722 Fat 53.3 g

Carbohydrates 3.6 g Sugar 2.3 g

Protein 54.1 g Cholesterol 204 mg

Fiber 1 g Net carbs 2.6 g

Spicy Adobo Pulled Pork

Preparation Time: 15 minutes

Cooking Time: 8 hours

Servings: 4

Ingredients:

2 lbs. pork

1 tbsp ground cumin

1 tbsp garlic, minced

7 oz chipotle peppers in adobo sauce

1 can chicken broth

Directions:

Put all listed items into the slow cooker and stir well. Cook within 8 hours on low.

Shred the meat using a fork. Stir well and serve.

Nutrition:

Calories 391 Fat 9.9 g Carbohydrates 10.1 g

Sugar 3.3 g Protein 62.7 g

Cholesterol 166 mg Fiber 5.9 g Net carbs 4.2 g

Tasty Pork Tacos

Preparation Time: 15 minutes
Cooking Time: 8 hours
Servings: 8
Ingredients:
2 lbs. pork tenderloin

2 tsp cayenne pepper

24 oz salsa

3 tsp garlic powder

2 tbsp ground cumin

2 tbsp chili powder

1 1/2 tsp salt

Directions:
Place pork tenderloin into the slow cooker.

Mix all rest of the ingredients except salsa in a small bowl. Rub spice mixture over pork tenderloin. Pour salsa on top of pork tenderloin.

Cook within 8 hours, low. Transfer the pork from slow cooker, and shred using a fork.

Return shredded pork into the slow cooker and stir well with salsa. Serve and enjoy.

Nutrition:

Calories 202 Fat 4.9 g

Carbohydrates 8 g Sugar 3.1 g

Protein 31.7 g Cholesterol 83 mg Fiber 2.4 g

Lamb Provençal

Preparation Time: 15 minutes
Cooking Time: 8 hours
Servings: 4
Ingredients:

2 racks lamb, approximately 2 pounds

1 Tablespoon olive oil

2 Tablespoons fresh rosemary, chopped

1 Tablespoon fresh thyme, chopped

4 garlic cloves, minced

1 teaspoon dry oregano

1 lemon, the zest

1 teaspoon minced fresh ginger

1 cup (Good) red wine

Salt and pepper to taste

Directions:

Preheat the crockpot on low.

In a pan, heat 1 tablespoon olive oil. Brown the meat for 2 minutes per side.

Mix remaining ingredients in a bowl.

Place the lamb in the crockpot, pour the remaining seasoning over the meat.

Cover, cook on low for 8 hours.

Nutrition:

Calories: 140 Carbs: 3g

Fat: 5g Protein: 21g

Greek Style Lamb Shanks

Preparation Time: 15 minutes
Cooking Time: 6 hours
Servings: 8
Ingredients:

3 Tablespoons butter

4 lamb shanks, approximately 1 pound each

2 Tablespoons olive oil

8-10 pearl onions

5 garlic cloves, minced

2 beef tomatoes, cubed

¼ cup of green olives

4 bay leaves

1 sprig fresh rosemary

1 teaspoon dry thyme

1 teaspoon ground cumin

1 cup fresh spinach

¾ cup hot water

½ cup red wine, Merlot or Cabernet

Salt and pepper to taste

Directions:

Liquify the butter in a pan, then cook the shanks on each side.

Remove, then add oil, onions, garlic. Cook for 3-4 minutes.

Add tomatoes, olives, spices, then stir well. Put the liquids and return the meat. Boil for 1 minute.

Transfer everything to the slow cooker.

Cover, cook on medium-high for 6 hours.

Nutrition:

Calories: 250 Carbs: 3g Fat: 16g Protein: 22g

Lamb with Mint & Green Beans

Preparation Time: 15 minutes

Cooking Time: 10 hours

Servings: 4

Ingredients:

½ t. salt – Himalayan pink

Freshly cracked black pepper

1 lamb leg – bone-in

2 tbsp. lard/ghee/tallow

4 garlic cloves

6 c. trimmed green beans

¼ freshly chopped mint/1-2 tbsp. dried mint

Directions:

Heat-up the slow cooker with a high setting.

Dry the lamb with some paper towels. Sprinkle with the pepper and salt. Grease a Dutch oven or similar large pot with the ghee/lard.

Sear the lamb until golden brown and set aside.

Remove the peels from the garlic and mince—dice up the mint. Arrange the seared meat into the slow cooker and give it a shake of the garlic and mint.

Secure the lid and program the cooker on the low-heat function (10 hrs.) or the high-function (6 hrs.).

After about four hours, switch the lamb out of the cooker. Toss in the green beans and return the lamb into the pot. Let the flavors mingle for about two more hours. The meat should be tender and the beans crispy. Serve and enjoy!

Nutrition:

Calories 525

Carbs 7.6 g

Protein 37.3 g

Fat 36.4 g

Delicious Balsamic Lamb Chops

Preparation Time: 15 minutes

Cooking Time: 6 hours

Servings: 6

Ingredients:

3.4 lbs. lamb chops, trimmed off

1/2 tsp ground black pepper

2 tbsp rosemary

2 tbsp balsamic vinegar

4 garlic cloves, minced

1 large onion, sliced

1/2 tsp salt

Directions:

Put the onion to the bottom of the slow cooker.

Place lamb chops on top of onions, add rosemary, vinegar, garlic, pepper, and salt.

Cook within 6 hours on low. Serve and enjoy.

Succulent Lamb

Preparation Time: 20 minutes

Cooking Time: 8 hours

Servings: 6

Ingredients:

¼ c. olive oil

1 (2 lb.) leg of lamb

1 tbsp. maple syrup

2 tbsp. whole grain mustard

4 thyme sprigs

6-7 mint leaves

¾ t. of each:

Dried rosemary

Garlic

Pepper & salt to taste

Directions:

Cut the string off of the lamb, then slice three slits over the top.

Cover the meat with the oil and the rub (mustard, pepper, salt, and maple syrup). Put the rosemary plus garlic into the slits.

Prepare on the low setting for seven hours. Garnish with the mint and thyme—Cook one more hour. Place on a platter and serve.

Nutrition:

Calories 414 Carbs 0.3 g Fat 35.2 g Protein 26.7 g

Tarragon Lamb & Beans

Preparation Time: 15 minutes

Cooking Time: 9 hours

Servings: 12

Ingredients:

4 (1 ½ lb.) lamb shanks

1 can (19 oz.) white beans/cannellini- for example

1 ½ c. peeled - diced carrot

2 thinly sliced garlic cloves

1 c. onion

¾ c. celery

2 t. dried tarragon

¼ t. freshly cracked black pepper

2 t. dried tarragon

1 can (28 oz.) diced tomatoes - not drained

Recommended: 7-quart slow cooker

Directions:

Discard all the fat from the lamb shanks. Pour the beans, cloves of garlic, chopped carrots, chopped celery, and onion in the cooker.

Put the shanks over the beans, and sprinkle with the salt, pepper, and tarragon. Empty the tomatoes over the lamb - including the juices—Cook, the lamb in the slow cooker on high for approximately one hour.

Reduce the temperature to the low setting and cook for nine hours or until the lamb is tender.

Remove, and set it aside. Empty the bean mixture through a colander over a bowl to reserve the liquid. Let the juices stand for five minutes and skim off the fat from the surface.

Return the bean mixture to the liquid in the slow cooker. Strip the lamb bones and throw the bones away.

Serve with the bean mixture and enjoy.

Nutrition:

Calories 353

Carbs 12.9 g

Fat 16.3 g

Protein 50.3 g

Apricot Pulled Pork

Preparation Time: 15 minutes

Cooking Time: 11 hours

Servings: 10

Ingredients:

3 pounds pork

1 cup barbecue sauce

6 ounces dried apricots

10 pounds apricot spread that does not contain any sugar

1 sweet onion

Directions:

Put the pork in the cooker. Add the barbecue, apricots, spread, and onions. Low cook for 11 hours.

Nutrition:

Calories 458 Fat 30 g Protein 33 g Carbs 15 g

Tantalizing Pork Chops with Cumin Butter and Garlic

Preparation Time: 15 minutes

Cooking Time: 4 hours

Servings: 4

Ingredients:

3.5 pounds of pork sirloin chops with the bone

½ cup of salsa

3 tablespoons of butter

5 tablespoons of lime juice

½ teaspoon of ground cumin

¾ teaspoon of garlic powder

¾ teaspoon of salt

¾ teaspoon of black pepper

Directions:

Combine the spices and season the pork chops.

Melt the butter in a saucepan and brown the pork chops for 3 minutes on each side.

Put it inside the slow cooker and pour the salsa over the top. Cook on high within 3-4 hours. Divide onto plates and serve.

Nutrition:

Calories: 364 Fat: 17 g Carbs: 3 g

Fiber: 0 g Protein: 51 g

New Mexico Carne Adovada

Preparation Time: 30 minutes
Cooking Time: 6 hours
Servings: 4
Ingredients:
2 tsp apple cider vinegar
1 tsp kosher salt
1 tsp ground coriander
1 tsp ground cumin
2 tsp dried Mexican oregano
6 garlic, sliced
1 onion, sliced
2 cups chicken stock
6 -8 ounces dried chilies, rinsed
3 pounds pork shoulder, cubes

Directions:
Put all the items in a pot, except the pork. Simmer it within 30-60 minutes, low.
Remove, then cooldown it within a few minutes.

Puree the batter in batches using a blender.

Put now the pork meat in a baking dish, covering it with the sauce. Chill within 1 to 2 days to marinate, stirring frequently.

Cook it in a slow cooker within 4 to 6 hours, low. Serve warm.

Nutrition:

Calories 120.2

Fat 5.3g

Carb 11.3g

Protein 8.0g

Smoky Pork with Cabbage

Preparation Time: 10 minutes

Cooking Time: 8 hours

Servings: 6

Ingredients:

lbs pastured pork roast

1/3 cup liquid smoke

1/2 cabbage head, chopped

1 cup water

1 tbsp kosher salt

Directions:

Rub pork with kosher salt and place into the slow cooker.

Pour liquid smoke over the pork. Add water.

Cover slow cooker with lid and cook on low for 7 hours.

Remove pork from slow cooker and add cabbage in the bottom of slow cooker.

Now place pork on top of the cabbage.

Cover again and cook for 1 hour more.

Shred pork with a fork and serves.

Nutrition:

Calories 484 Fat 21.5 g

Carbohydrates 3.5 g

Sugar 1.9 g Protein 65.4 g

Cholesterol 195 mg

Simple Roasted Pork Shoulder

Preparation Time: 10 minutes

Cooking Time: 9 hours

Servings: 8

Ingredients:

lbs pork shoulder

1 tsp garlic powder

1/2 cup water

1/2 tsp black pepper

1/2 tsp sea salt

Directions:

Season pork with garlic powder, pepper, and salt and place in slow cooker. Add water.

Cover slow cooker with lid and cook on high for 1 hour then turn heat to low and cook for 8 hours.

Remove meat from slow cooker and shred using a fork. Serve and enjoy.

Flavors Pork Chops

Preparation Time: 10 minutes
Cooking Time: 4 hours
Servings: 4
Ingredients:
pork chops
2 garlic cloves, minced
1 cup chicken broth
1 tbsp poultry seasoning
1/4 cup olive oil
Pepper and salt
Directions:
In a bowl, whisk together olive oil, poultry seasoning, garlic, broth, pepper, and salt.
Pour olive oil mixture into the slow cooker then place pork chops into the slow cooker.
Cover slow cooker with lid and cook on high for 4 hours.
Serve and enjoy.
Nutrition:

Calories 386

Fat 32.9 g

Carbohydrates 2.9 g

Sugar 0.7 g

Protein 19.7 g

Pork Loin with Peanut Sauce

Preparation Time: 10 minutes
Cooking Time: 8 hours
Servings: 8
Ingredients:

2 pounds pork tenderloin

2 tablespoons olive oil

1 teaspoon salt

1 teaspoon black pepper

2 cups cabbage, shredded

1 cup chicken stock

½ cup peanut butter

¼ cup soy sauce

1 tablespoon rice vinegar

1 tablespoon crushed red pepper flakes

1 tablespoon cayenne pepper sauce

2 cloves garlic crushed and minced

½ cup peanuts, chopped

1 tablespoon fresh lemongrass, chopped

Directions:

Brush the tenderloin with olive oil and season it with salt and black pepper.

Arrange the tenderloin and cabbage in a slow cooker.

In a bowl, combine the chicken stock, peanut butter, soy sauce, rice vinegar, crushed red pepper flakes, cayenne pepper sauce, and garlic. Whisk them together and pour the sauce into the slow cooker. Stir gently to distribute the sauce.

Sprinkle in the peanuts and lemongrass.

Cover and cook on low for 8 hours.

Nutrition:

Calories 427.4, Total Fat 25.5 g,

Saturated Fat 4.9 g, Total Carbs 6.9 g,

Approx. Net Carbs: 5 g, Dietary Fiber 2.3 g